INTRODUCTION

Dengue as a Global Threat

Dengue is a disease caused by four closely related viruses known as dengue virus -1 through -4 (DENV1-DENV4). A fifth serotype (DENV5) was discovered from a serological sample from 2007 but is not published. Dengue fever is a disease that became prevalent in tropics during the great shipping industry expansion in the 18th and 19th centuries [4]. The principle arthropod vectors of dengue virus, the Aedes aegypti and Aedes albopictus mosquitoes, determine the geographic distribution of the disease. Approximately 40% of the world's population (2.5 billion people) live in a region at risk of dengue [2]. Dengue is typically spread throughout the tropical and subtropical latitudes, but has demonstrated the ability to spread to new areas, such as Europe, Croatia, the United States, and Portuguese islands [2]. Based on the morbidity of dengue infection and the widespread presence of its vectors, DENV is considered the most important arbovirus (arthropod-borne virus) in the world [1]–[3]. Vector control is the primary means of stopping an outbreak and ending the disease transmission cycle.

Dengue Pathology

Dengue is transmitted through the bite of an infected female mosquito during its blood meal [5]. Humans are a dead-end host and the infection is not transmissible between humans. A noninfected Aedes mosquito can become infected through a blood meal on an infected human. After 4-10 days post-infection, a mosquito is an infectious vector for the remainder of its life [2]. The severity of an individual's infection depends largely on the history of infection and is characterized by the three clinical categories –

1

dengue fever, dengue hemorrhagic fever (DHF) or dengue shock syndrome (DSS). Primary infection may be asymptomatic or lead to classic dengue fever. Secondary infections may lead to the serious conditions of DHF or DSS [1].

The World Health Organization estimates that 50-100 million people are infected with dengue each year. Due to the lack in accurate and timely reporting and the absence of adequate medical facilities in endemic regions, other sources, such as the Centers for Disease Control (CDC) place this estimate as high as 400 million annual infections [3]. Classic dengue fever is the predominant syndrome. DHF accounts for over 500 thousand reported cases and there are over 22 thousand deaths annually [2].

Classic dengue fever is also known as "breakbone fever", and was first described by Benjamin Rush during an outbreak in Philadelphia in 1780 [5]. Dengue fever begins after a 5-8 day incubation period with the abrupt onset of fever (103-106^{0}F) and headache (Figure 1). In the first day or two of fever, the face flushes and a generalized macular rash becomes evident. Between days 4-6, symptoms include nausea, vomiting, anorexia, and swollen lymph nodes (lymphadenopathy). The fever typically lasts 4-6 days and often culminates with a secondary maculopapular rash. The level of viremia generally coincides with fever.

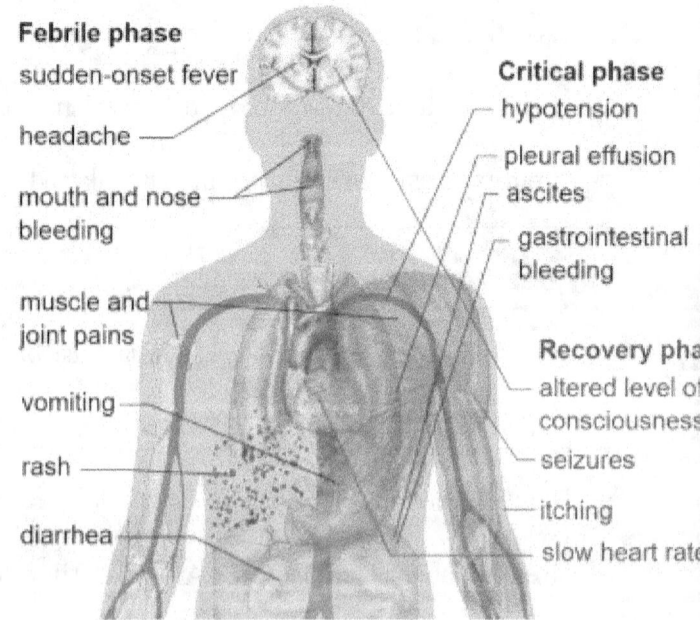

Figure 1. Symptoms of dengue fever. Public domain im via Wikimedia Commons.

2

Dengue hemorrhagic fever (DHF) and dengue shock syndrome (DSS) are severe

forms of dengue infection that can lead to death. DHF and DSS are common in areas

with multiple endemic DENV serotypes. These serious illnesses begin with typical

dengue fever. Severe symptoms follow 2-5 days later with petechiae, bruising, and large

spontaneous bruising (ecchymosis).

Table 1. World Health Organization grades of dengue fever (DF), hemorrhagic fever (DHF), or shock (DSS) [6].

Grade of disease	Disease type	Signs and Symptoms
I	DF	Fever accompanied by nonspecific constitutional symptoms with a positive tourniquet test as the only hemorrhagic manifestation
II	DHF	Same as grade I, except with spontaneous hemorrhagic manifestations
III	DSS	Circulatory failure manifested by rapid, weak pulse with narrowing of the pulse pressure (<20 mmHg) or hypotension
IV	DSS	Profound shock with undetectable blood pressure and pulse

DHF and DSS are typically found in cases of secondary infection with a DENV

serotype different from that of primary infection. These clinical developments are

brought on by an immunological phenomenon called antibody dependent enhancement

(ADE). For example, following a successful adaptive immune response to primary

DENV1 infection, antibodies are created which recognize DENV1 epitopes and can assist

only in the neutralization DENV1. During a secondary infection with DENV2, the

circulating antibodies that recognize DENV1 attach to the unfamiliar DENV2 particles

and facilitate endocytosis by macrophages by means of the cognate (DENV-recognizing)

receptors. However, the circulating antibodies only weakly activate the cellular defenses and the virus will still undergo replication. Additionally, the DENV1 antibodies bound to DENV2 particles will be able to bind and enter cells through the Fc (constant) receptors which are ubiquitously expressed. This additional infectious pathway greatly contributes to the progressive symptoms of severe dengue (DHF/DSS).

Dengue Threatens DOD Operations

The United States has military and civilian personnel stationed in many countries around the world. Some of these locations are in regions where Dengue is endemic and a growing threat to the human population [3]. Although dengue fever is uncommon among US citizens, dengue is a top priority for health and medical services in endemic areas. Dengue has caused illness in US military personnel in every major conflict since the Spanish American War, excluding the recent Iraq and Afghanistan campaigns [7]. From the 1960s and through the 1990s, dengue infections were seen often in US servicemembers in Vietnam, the Philippines, Somalia, and Haiti. In 1942, a dengue outbreak effected 80% of a single unit stationed in the Australian North Territory [7]. Although the total number of cases in this outbreak was not documented, it casts a dark shadow in the potential for entire military units to be rendered incapable of performing their mission. In 1944, over 24 thousand troops in New Guinea and approximately 20 thousand in the Marshall Islands were confirmed to have dengue. Throughout WWII, seventeen US bases were impacted by dengue [7].

Dengue is a historic problem within the continental United States. Between 1977 and 1987, 1655 suspected cases of dengue were observed in the southern states, 345 of which were confirmed by serological tests. These cases occurred long after dengue was

4

eliminated from the southern US in the 1920s. This example shows that the potential for reintroduction of dengue still exists. The most recent outbreaks of DENV occurred in Hawaii (2001), Texas (2005), and Florida (2014) [3].

Dengue as a Potential Bioterrorism Agent

DENV is classified as a Biosafety Level 2 (BL-2) virus. Some fear that biological agents could be used to contaminate water supplies. DENV is not found naturally in water supplies and must infect living cells to replicate. DENV is expected to survive in untreated water for short periods but not is not expected to survive common water treatment methods [8]. In this suspended form, DENV would not be infectious and requires parenteral transmission. Dengue is only infectious through parenteral transmission which greatly limits the potential for non-vector dissemination. Dengue does not exhibit rapid or morbid common in biowarfare agents and is not lethal unless severe shock or other complications are involved.

Challenges to Dengue Therapeutics

The design and implementation of a dengue vaccine is complicated by numerous factors. First, the candidate vaccine must provide equal and lasting immune responses against all DENV serotypes. This requires a tetravalent vaccine to address DENV1-4, and a pentavalent vaccine if the novel DENV5 is considered. This vaccine would also need to solicit neutralizing antibodies regardless of the individuals existing immune status to DENV [6]. A second challenge is that there is not a validated correlate of protection. Since the mechanism of DENV infection is not completely understood, the required antibody titers and impact of additional immunological pathways require further study [9]. Third, an animal model does not exist which recapitulates both the disease outcome and a predictive immune response in humans. Currently, mouse and non-human primate (NHP) models are used to evaluate vaccine candidates. The mouse model requires modification of the viral genome to present clinical disease and may not be indicative of efficacy in humans. The NHP model does not present clinical disease but does demonstrate viremia. Possibly due to these factors, discordance is occasionally observed between preclinical and clinical trials [10].

Vaccines development is complicated by small mutations in DENV serotypes. One common mechanism of each DENV serotype and flaviviruses in general is the action of RNA-dependent RNA polymerase (RdRp). This enzyme catalyzes the replication of RNA from the ss(+)RNA strand [11], [12]. Novartis developed an adenosine nucleoside inhibitor (NITD008) which directly inhibits the RdRp activity of DENV in vitro and in vivo. NITD008 is an adenosine analog with several substitutions; a carbon for N-7 of the purine and an acetylene at the 2' position of ribose [12]. Potential may exist for AgNP to inhibit DENV by binding to exposed disulfide motifs within DENV RdRp [11].

Nanoparticles as an Antiviral Treatment

Nanoparticle therapeutics are in their infancy and there are currently no FDA approved nanotherapudics [13]. Several studies demonstrate the systemic effects of silver nanoparticles through various routes of exposure [14]–[17]. In a mouse model, inhalational and gastrointestinal exposure (1-3 months) to AgNP (20nm, citrate stabilized) did not show severe systemic toxicity but intravenous exposure has potential to suppress the functional immune system in a dose-dependent manner (0.0082-6 mg/mL)

6

[15]. Research also suggests that NP have potential to penetrate the blood-brain barrier (BBB) through intravenous and intraperitoneal exposure at high doses (25-100 mg/kg) [14].

These and similar studies offer unique insight to in vivo actions of AgNP but they do not offer broad applicability outside the structure of the research. Published research involving AgNP does not consistently provide full characterization of the administered silver with respect to silver ion content, particle agglomeration, particle size distribution, surface coatings, or presence of synthesis byproducts. Since these additional factors play a critical role in AgNP biocompatibility and in vivo response, such omissions reduce the transferability of those data. Above certain concentrations (often $>100\mu g/mL$), AgNPs may exhibit genotoxic and cytotoxic effects in human tissue culture. The possibility that this effect is due to higher concentration of silver ions must be considered. This can lead to DNA damage, chromosomal aberrations, and cell death [18]. If AgNP are to be utilized in clinical settings, the applied concentration must be well characterized under in vivo applications and remain under the cytotoxic levels.

LITERATURE REVIEW

Dengue Virus Summary

DENV is a member of the Flavivirus family, as is the yellow fever virus (the family's prototype), West Nile, Japanese encephalitis virus, and many others. DENV is also categorized as a Group IV ss(+)RNA virus under the Baltimore Classification. Based on serological studies, five serotypes of DENV (DENV1-5) are known to exist [19], [20]. While DENV1-4 are in common circulation, DENV5 is known only to exist in a single outbreak in Malaysia, presents challenges for the future of DENV vaccines and treatments. Many scientists are skeptical about the serological independence of DENV5 and feel more research is necessary to determine if it is not a mutant of another DENV serotype [21]. These distinct serotypes present conserved structural and non-structural proteins although the genome identity between serotypes ranges from 23-73% [22], [23]. DENV virions exist in one of four stages of maturation. Only one of the four stages is infectious and considered mature. The mature virions exist in the extracellular environment while the three immature virion forms are primarily found intracellularly.

A mature DENV virion is composed of envelope proteins surrounding a nucleocapsid core which contains the viral genome. The genome consists of a single, positive-sense strand of RNA, approximately 10.7kb in length. The vRNA is translated into a single polyprotein. Viral and host proteases cleave this into three structural (C, prM, E) and seven non-structural (NS1-NS2A-NS2B-NS3-NS4A-NS4B-NS5) proteins. The genome is surrounded by an icosahedral nucleocapsid C (capsid) protein approximately 30nm in diameter [5]. The nucleocapsid is disordered and associated with the vRNA in an overlapping region [24]. This core is surrounded by a lipid bilayer then a well-organized icosahedral envelope which consists of E-prM protein heterodimeric complexes [5], [25].

DENV successfully grows in many cells lines from vertebrate and invertebrate hosts, but the most common are the C6/36 (ATCC® CRL-1660™) derived from the Aedes albopictus mosquito and the Cercopithecus aethiops (African green monkey) kidney epithelial (Vero) cell lineage [5], [26]. Selection of the C6/36 cells for DENV

8

research is often preferable since they originate from the virus host. The titer of DENV isolated from C6/36 cell propagation tends to higher and express less mutations than

isolates from Vero cells propagation [26]. However, as an invertebrate cell line, the utilization of C6/36 cells requires growth at 28°C. Since this was a condition not supported at the researcher's laboratory facility, Vero cells were selected as a suitable cell line for virus propagation and additional assays.

Dengue Virus Binding and Entry

Dengue virus binds to mammalian cells through a wide range of cell-surface receptors and co-receptors. Among the known DENV receptors, heparin sulfate (Vero cells), DC-SIGN, and the mannose receptor (macrophages) appear to play a critical role [27]–[29]. In the event of antibody-dependent enhancement, the ubiquitous Fc receptor enhances DENV infection by binding anti-DENV antibodies and providing another entry pathway. The DENV E protein (envelope glycoprotein) is the central epitope during binding. Once bound to the cell, DENV is trafficked in a diffusive manner along the cell surface until reaching a pre-existing clathrin-coated pit [30]. Dengue entry into mammalian cells may occur through multiple mechanisms, dominated by clathrin-mediated endocytosis and macropinocytosis [31], [32].

In the dominant case of clathrin-mediated endocytosis, DENV is internalized when the clathrin-coated pit invaginates and surrounds the particle. Now considered an endosome, the pH is lowered through action of proton pumps. The acidic pH causes a conformational change in the E protein below pH 6.2, causing it to become spiked in appearance. The hydrophobic tips of the spiked envelope proteins penetrate and fuse with the endosomal membrane, releasing the DENV genome into the cytoplasm.

Silver Nanoparticles as Antiviral Agents

During the course of this research, the interaction of AgNP with 10 virus species were identified (Table 2). Each study concluded that AgNP inhibited the course of that particular virus replication cycle under certain conditions. The mechanism of inhibition was not consistent between all viruses and some mechanisms are still unknown. One common conclusion was that inhibitory mechanisms occurred early in the replication cycle, most commonly inhibiting the binding and entry of a virion into a host cell.

Table 2. Existing research silver nanoparticles as antiviral treatments. Organized by Baltimore Classification. **DENV is utilized for the first time in this research.

I dsDNA	II ssDNA	III dsRNA	IV ss(+)RNA	V ss(-)RNA	VI ssRNA-RT	VII dsDNA-RT
Vaccinia [33] Monkeypox [34] HSV2 [35] Adenovirus			**DENV	H1N1 [36] H3N2 [37] TCRV [38] RSV [39]	HIV-1 [40]–[43]	HBV [44]

Common experimental conditions which led to successful inhibition include:

- Antiviral activity dependence on AgNP size

- AgNP diameters between 8-25nm

- AgNP concentrations between 8-50µg/mL

- Tangential flow filtration (TFF) for AgNP size selection and silver ion removal

- AgNP which are naked or capped or stabilized with citrate, polyethylene glycol (PEG), or polyvinylpyrrolidone

Vaccinia virus (VACV)

Silver Nanoparticles demonstrated cytoprotective and virucidal effects during VACV infection of Vero cells [33], [43]. Adsorption of VACV was not prevented when Vero cells were pretreated with AgNP (11nm, 8-128μg/mL), as determined by plaque assay. The entry of vaccinia virus into Vero cells is inhibited by AgNP at values above 48μg/mL as determined by a β-gal (beta galactosidase) assay under the control of a constitutively active promoter. Through confocal microscopy quantification, VACV entry was inhibited when pretreated $\geq$ 16μg/mL. VACV is an enveloped dsDNA virus that replicated entirely in the cytoplasm. VACV is in the family Poxviridae and contains both a large genome (~190kbp) and large virion (~300nm). VACV enters host cells through macropinocytosis and direct fusion.

Monkeypox virus (MPV)

MPV infection of Vero cells was inhibited by 10nm polysaccharide-coated AgNP [34]. AgNP in diameters of 10-80nm, concentrations from 12.5-100μg/mL, and either polysaccharide coated or naked were tested against MPV in plaque reduction assays. Only the 10nm PS-coated AgNP reduced mean PFU below control ($P \leq 0.05$). This result is similar to HIV-1 studies with AgNP where smaller particles (1-10nm) provided the best antiviral activity. Rogers, et al. suggest the small particles effectively bind to viral epitopes and block the binding complex between virus and cell surface receptors and co-receptors. Another conclusion of this research was that the mechanism of

11

inhibition is unknown but may "involve blocking of MPV to host cells, disruption of host cell biochemical pathways, or both" [34]. MPV is similar to VACV in size and replication cycle.

Herpes simplex virus (HSV)

AgNP of unspecified diameter and concentration reportedly inhibit HBV2 in Vero cells. Sopova et al. described in the Russian journal (not translated to English) that "silver nanopowders" significantly reduced viral progeny in vitro. HSV is an enveloped dsDNA virus (152kbp) that enters host cells through fusion.

Adenovirus type 3 (ADV3)

Adenoviruses are non-enveloped dsDNA viruses with a diameter of 70–90 nm. ADV3 infection of HeLa cells was inhibited by AgNP (11.4 ± 6.2nm) in concentrations from 3.125-50µg/mL [45]. Cytopathic effects were observed in in HeLa cells when AgNP concentrations exceeded 50µg/mL as seen in similar experiments. Unlike most AgNP antiviral experiments which treat cells and virus for 1 hour, Chen et al. treated for 2 hours. ADV3 that was treated with 50µg/mL AgNP for 30 minutes experienced conformational changes in the virion structure. Treatment for 90 and 120 minutes created dramatic damage to the virion. Unfortunately, the researchers did not mention whether their AgNP colloid contained significant levels of silver ions, the most likely cause of ADV3 damage.

Influenza A (H1N1 and H3N2 IFV)

H1N1 and H3N2 influenza A infection of Madin-Darby Canine Kidney epithelial (MDCK) cells was inhibited by non-coated AgNP [36], [37]. AgNP in these studies were

12

characterized in the range of 5-120nm (10nm mean). This study found that when H1N1 or H3N2 IFV were pretreated for 2 hours with AgNP concentrations of 12.5-50μg/mL, the viability of MDCK cells was significantly increased ($P<0.01$). When virus was incubated with AgNP (50μg/mL) for 30-120 minutes, the IFV experienced structural damage. Damage was observed even when there did not appear to be AgNP bound to virions, indicating damage through silver ions. These studies recognized the potential significance of silver ions in an antiviral mechanism but did not present data on ion content in their colloid or any methods used to remove silver ions during experimentation.

Tacaribe virus (TCRV)

Tacaribe virus infection of Vero cells was inhibited by AgNP of varying size and coating [38]. AgNP (10nm and 25nm) that were either naked or polysaccharide-coated significantly inhibited viral progeny ($P<0.05$). AgNP concentrations above 50μg/mL were determined to exhibit cytopathic effect. Unlike other AgNP antiviral studies, TCRV experienced enhanced uptake into Vero cells when in complex with 10nm non-coated AgNP (50μg/mL). Replication was inhibited after entry to the cell by an unknown mechanism.

Respiratory syncytial virus (RSV)

RSV infection of HEp-2 cells was reduced by 44% after RSV pretreatment with poly(N-vinyl-2-pyrrolidone) (PVP) coated AgNP. These functionalized AgNP exhibited low cytotoxicity at low concentrations.

Human immunodeficiency virus (HIV-1)

Several studies have determined that HIV-1 (or HIV-1 pseudotyped virus [43]) binding and entry to host cells can be inhibited by AgNP pretreatment [40]–[43]. Common conclusions indicate that AgNP ($\leq$25nm) bind to the glycoprotein 120 (gp120) knobs of the HIV-1 envelope but a 1-10nm diameter is optimal [42]. This binding event blocks the formation of the gp120-CD4 complex and inhibits cell fusion. One study determined that the use of AgNP and neutralizing antibodies had an additive inhibitory effect against cell-associated HIV-1 [41].

Hepatitis B (HBV)

AgNP (10nm & 50nm, uncoated) inhibit hepatitis B virus replication in HepAD38 cells [44]. The suggested mechanism of inhibition is the direct interaction between AgNP and the HBV dsDNA or virion. Lu et al. determined through TEM that the 10nm particles were able to bind directly to the HBV virion. AgNP had little effect on HBV circular DNA but inhibited the formation of HBV intracellular RNA. HBV is an enveloped dsDNA virus with a reverse transcription intermediate (dsDNA-RT). HBV is generally spherical and 42nm in diameter (similar to DENV, 50nm) but pleomorphic forms exist including filamentous and spheres without a nucleocapsid core.

Silver Ions

It is important for AgNP research to differentiate between effects of silver nanoparticles and silver ions. AgNP are widely viewed as antimicrobial, but it may actually be the silver ions present in the colloid that impart protective effects. Silver ions (Ag^+) are known to possess antibacterial effects by the mechanism is not fully

14

understood. Silver ions are also cytotoxic at much lower concentrations than ion-free AgNP colloids. Potential in-vivo treatments must utilize well-characterized silver colloids to ensure ion levels are safe. Silver ions interact with thiol groups in enzymes and proteins, altering their intended conformation and function [46]. Ions released from silver nanoparticle colloids is known to inactivate enterobacter aerogenes-specific bacteriophage (UZ1). Silver ions in the form of silver nitrate ($AgNO_3$) also inactivated the MS2 and T2 phages and implicated in the inactivation of numerous other viruses [34], [47], [48]. The bactericidal effect of silver ions are well known and provide the antibacterial properties of silver used in medical dressings, surgical tools, and many commercial products [49].

Silver Nanoparticle Selection

The increased attention of potential AgNP antiviral properties led to numerous studies regarding the influence of AgNP size, concentration, surface modification, and morphology on their viralcidal or cytoprotective effects [34]–[43]. Several reports indicate that uncoated, spherical AgNPs of approximately 10-20nm in diameter are the most effective at preventing viral infection in a variety of cell lines while avoiding significant host cell cytotoxicity [34], [38], [42]. Such particles commonly exhibit non-cytotoxic antiviral effects at concentrations ≤50μg/mL.

Stabilizing AgNP with citrate (1%) prevents aggregation and improves particle suspension in a colloid. Citrate stabilizes the AgNP by creating an electrostatic barrier in weak complex with the particles. Citrate is easily displaced which permits unhindered binding between AgNP and ligands such as sulfides on viral envelopes [50].

MATERIALS AND METHODS

Overview

Research was conducted in three phases: characterization, fluorescence, and analysis. First, the key components of the research were characterized (Vero cells, AgNP, and DENV2). Vero cells were passaged numerous times to ensure they were free of foreign contamination and their growth curve was determined at 24 hour intervals. The silver nanoparticles used in this research were analyzed for size distribution, colloid concentration, and aggregation. DENV2 was propagated in Vero cells and titrated by plaque assay and flow cytometry. Second, the effect of AgNP, DENV, and DENV-AgNP were explored through immunofluorescence binding assays. The impact of AgNP on DENV binding to Vero cells constituted the endpoint assay of this research. Third, the fluorescent images were processed and analyzed to determine the effect of AgNP on DENV binding to Vero cells.

Vero Cells

Vero 76 cells (CRL-1587, ATCC) are African green monkey kidney epithelial cells. Vero cells are commonly used in microbiology, molecular and cell biology research when a continuous mammalian cell line is required [51]. Vero cells are anchorage-dependent and susceptible to a wide range of viral infection, thus permitting the study of viral infection through plaque reduction assays and other common analytical techniques [51]. Vero cells have been used extensively with DENV and are a proven model for DENV experimentation [5], [26], [52].

16

To reliably perform experiments in cell culture with repeatable results, it is important to accurately predict the cell population at various points. Vero cell growth is commonly reported to double in each 24h period until day 6, when the growth is significantly slower [53]. Growth rates over 96h for the particular Vero cells used in this research exhibited a 12h stabilization period of attachment and 80% growth every 24h period over 96h (Figure 2) as determined by cell counting using the hemacytometer method (described below).

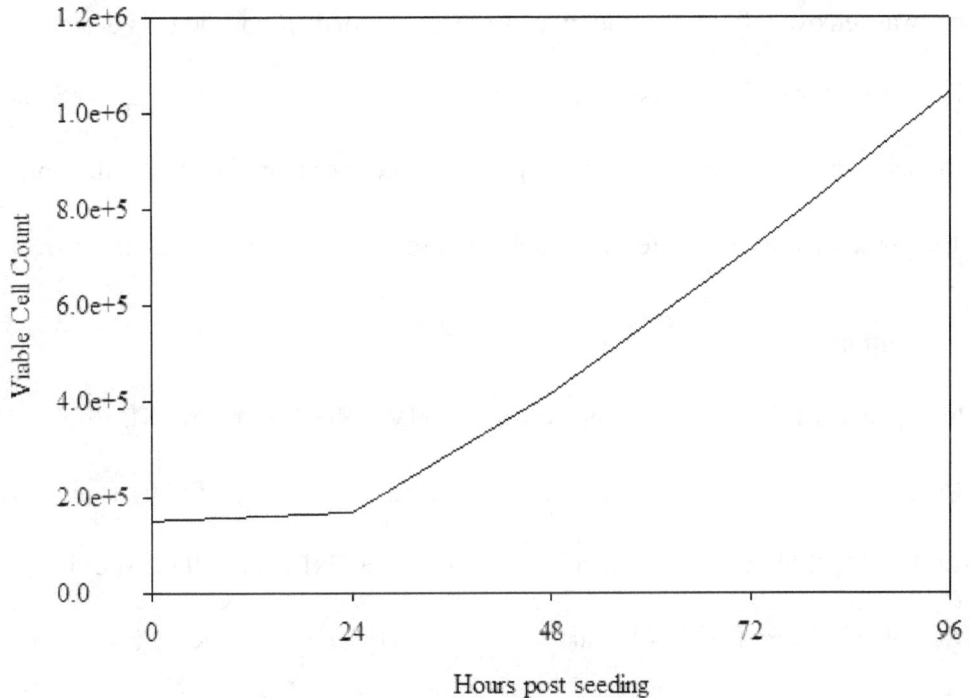

Figure 2. Vero cell 96-hour growth curve

Cell Line Maintenance

Vero 76 (ATCC® CRL-1587™) cells were maintained according to established protocols [51], [54]. Cells were maintained in DMEM/High Glucose (HyClone®) supplemented with 10% heat-inactivated Fetal Bovine Serum and 1% Penicillin/Streptomycin (Sigma®, 10k U/mL penicillin and 10mg/mL streptomycin in

0.9% NaCl). During subculture procedures, cell count and viability was performed by the Trypan Blue exclusion test using a hemacytometer, described below. This permitted a high consistency in cell growth timelines and cell survival. A cell growth curve (Figure 2) was established as a baseline for experiments influencing cellular growth rates and to provide greater consistency and predictability when preparing for experiments.

Five 60mm petri dishes were seeded with Vero cells at a density of $15x10^4$ per dish, as determined by the hemacytometer method of cell counting. At 24 hour intervals, one culture was removed from incubation and processed for cell counting as described below. The slow growth in the first 24 hours is typical since the cells take approximately 12 hours to stabilize in the media, and undergo the process of adhesion to the dish prior to entering the phase of growth where they double approximately every 24 hours [53].

Virus Propagation

Propagation of Dengue virus serotype 2 (DENV2-NGC) (Dr. Eric M. Vela, Battelle Research Center) was performed in Vero 76 cells. The titer of virus stock was approximately 10^6 PFU/mL. Vero 76 cells were seeded at $2x10^6$ in 100 mm petri dishes in DMEM/High Glucose (HyClone®) supplemented with 10% heat-inactivated Fetal Bovine Serum and 1% Penicillin/Streptomycin (Sigma®, 10k U/mL penicillin and 10mg/mL streptomycin in 0.9% NaCl). The cells were incubated at 37°C and 5% CO_2 until they reached a confluency of approximately 90% then infected with DENV2 for 5-6 days, which was prior to significant cytopathic effects as observed through a light microscope. Previous research has demonstrated that the presence of serum in the growth media during DENV propagation does not inhibit the titer yield but is necessary for proper cell maintenance in culture [55]. The cells were then detached from the growth surface with Trypsin and centrifuged at 3200 rpm (2136x g) at 4°C for 10 minutes to eliminate cell debris. Immature (non-infectious) isoforms of DENV are primarily intracellular and captured in the pellet following centrifugation. The virus recovered from the supernatant contain primarily mature (infectious) DENV although the various isoforms can never be isolated with 100% efficiency. The supernatant was aliquoted and stored at −80°C until use. Virus stock was filtered before use using 0.22μm filter membranes (EMD Millipore).

Virus Quantification by Flow Cytometry

Dengue virus titers were determined by plaque assay in confluent monolayers of Vero 76 cells grown in 6-well plates. Vero 76 cells were inoculated with ten-fold serial dilutions when monolayers reached 80 to 90% confluence. After 2 hours of viral adsorption, the monolayers were overlaid with 2 ml of Opti-MEM GlutaMAX (Life Technologies Inc.) containing 2% Methyl-cellulose (Acros Organics) and 0.5% fetal bovine serum. The cultures were incubated at 37 °C for 5-6 days and then counted for plaque formation after fixation with 4% paraformaldehyde and staining with 1% crystal violet solution (Sigma). Additionally viral titers were also determined using flow cytometry as described by Medina et al [26]. Briefly, Vero cells grown in 24-well plates at a density of $1.25x10^5$ per well 24 hours prior to infection were infected with ten-fold serial dilutions of DENV2 diluted in Opti-MEM. After incubating one hour with gentle rocking every 15 minutes, the supernatant was aspirated and overlaid with 1ml of 2% methyl cellulose and incubated at 37 °C for 24 hours. Next day, infected monolayers

19

were trypsinized, fixed, blocked for unspecific binding and then stained with DENV2 monoclonal antibody 4G2 (Millipore). These antibodies are directed to the E protein of the dengue virus and are capable of specifically neutralizing DENV2 serotype. Because these antibodies are not fluorescent tagged, the cells were stained with fluorescein isothiocyanate (FITC) conjugated secondary antibodies (Biolegend) and analyzed using Accuri C6 flow cytometer. Final viral titers were calculated as infectious units (IU)/ml.

Silver Nanoparticle Synthesis and Filtration

AgNPs were synthesized by the reduction of 0.4% w/v (~0.024 M) silver nitrate (AgNO$_3$, MW=169.87, Sigma-Aldrich) with 0.5% w/v (~0.132 M) sodium borohydride (NaBH$_4$, MW=37.83, Sigma-Aldrich) in an aqueous matrix, stabilized by 1.0% w/v (~0.034 M) trisodium citrate dihydrate (Na$_3$C$_6$H$_5$O$_7$·2H$_2$O, MW=294.10, Fluka). In a dark chemical fume hood, 50mL of 4°C de-ionized water and 1.25mL of 0.4% silver nitrate were combined and mixed with a magnetic stirrer for 1 minute. 500uL of 0.5% sodium borohydride was rapidly added to the sidewall of the solution while mixing vigorously for 1 minute. After 1 minute, 200uL of 1% sodium citrate was added and continuously stirred for an additional 1 minute. The solution was placed in a foil covered 50 mL conical tube and kept stored at 4°C until use.

This synthesis results in a colloid containing spherical AgNPs with a mean diameter of 8nm. This method also results in trace amounts of non-reduced silver ions following the formation of AgNPs. Silver ions were removed through tangential flow filtration.

Tangential flow filtration (TFF) was employed to size-select AgNPs for viral inhibition studies. Typically reserved for biological separations, TFF operates on the continuous recirculation of a solution containing an analyte of interest across a porous membrane (Figure 3). As a solution or colloid is passed over the membrane, larger components are retained by the filter membrane and kept within the recirculation tubing (e.g. gray spheres in Figure 3) while constituents smaller than the filter pores are passed through the membrane and collected in a dilute filtrate (e.g. blue spheres in Figure 3).

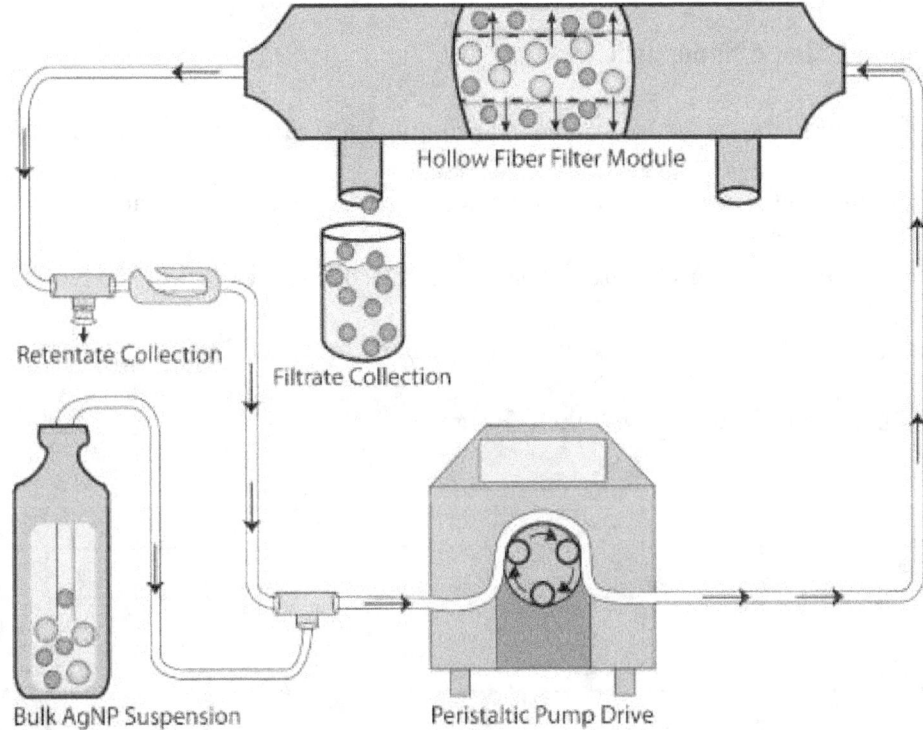

Figure 3. Schematic depicting a typical TFF set-up for the filtration of colloidal AgNPs. Gray and blue spheres represent AgNPs larger and smaller than the filter membrane pores, respectively.

By employing filters of varying pore size, AgNPs were size-selected for diameters of approximately 5-20nm (8nm average) and concentrated by removing excess solvent using membranes with ultrafine pore sizes (e.g., 5nm in diameter). The TFF process resulted in a significantly concentrated colloid (i.e., 10mL of AgNPs at a concentration of 1,000µg/mL or higher) that can be utilized to create viral inhibition titers free of excess reagents, which might interfere with the interpretation of the antiviral mechanism exhibited by AgNPs.

The concentration of nanosilver in the AgNP titers and TFF-obtained colloid was determined spectrophotometrically using inductively coupled plasma optical emission spectroscopy (ICP-OES).

Characterization of Silver Nanoparticles

AgNP characteristics monitored in this research include, size and size distribution, colloid concentration, zeta potential, silver ion content, and the presence of stabilizing compounds (i.e. citrate). The AgNP colloid utilized for the binding inhibition study were citrate stabilized and exhibited an average hydrodynamic diameter of 23.5nm $\pm$0.95nm (DLS, Figure 17), and a UV-Vis (peak 400nm, Figure 4).

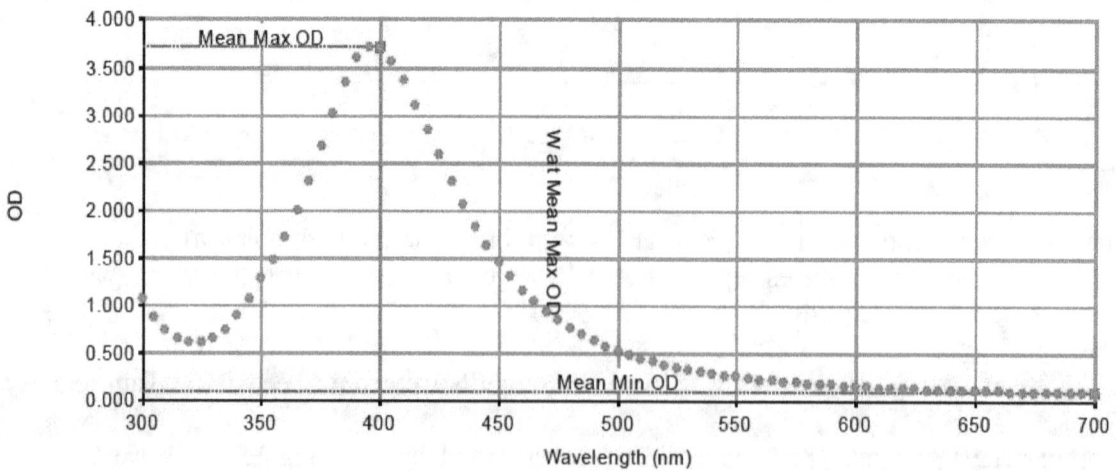

Figure 4. UV-Vis spectra for the AgNP colloid utilized in binding inhibition assay.

Characterization of nanoparticles was conducted at the Air Force Research

Laboratory RHDJ Biomolecular Interaction of Nanomaterials (BIN) facility at Wright

Patterson Air Force Base. Following synthesis and prior to use, nanoparticles were

characterized using the following work flow (Figure 5):

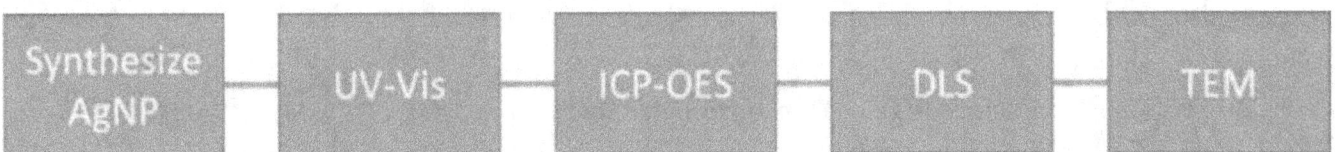

Figure 5. Work flow for AgNP characterization

- UV-Vis – Ultraviolet–visible spectroscopy (size/agglomeration, Figure 6A),

- DLS – Dynamic light scattering (size, zeta potential, Figure 6B)

- ICP-OES – Inductively coupled plasma optical emission spectrometry (concentration)

- TEM – Transmission electron microscopy (visualization, size).

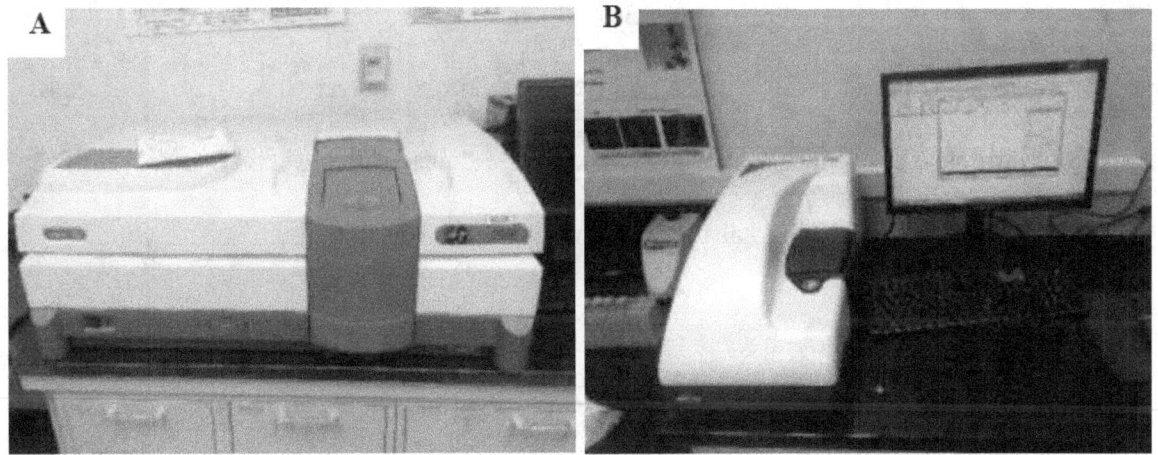

Figure 6. Nanoparticle characterization equipment. (A) Varian Cary 5000 UV-Vis, (B) Malvern Zetasizer Nano ZS.

AgNP-DENV2 Treatment

Silver nanoparticles were incubated with DENV2 at room temperature in various concentrations (10, 25, 50, 100μg/mL) for one hour prior to Vero cell infection. This pre-treatment timeline was chosen in order to allow stable binding between DENV2 and the AgNP.

Trypan Blue Exclusion Test (Hemacytometer method)

Trypan Blue staining was performed during cell culture to ensure continued viability of the Vero cells between passages. Trypan Blue staining was also performed to support the results of MTT assays (cell viability). After centrifugation, cells were suspended in DMEM and titurated thoroughly. A hemacytometer was cleaned with 70% ethanol and a 20mm glass coverslip was placed over the viewing grid. 50μL of the cell suspension was added to 100μL Trypan Blue stain in a 0.5mL centrifuge tube and titurated thoroughly. This 50:100 ratio provided a dilution factor of 3. The cell-stain mixture was pipetted into the loading channel until the viewing grid was full (approximately 10μL). Viable cells exclude the stain and appear white while dead cells take up the stain and appear blue. Eight grids were counted (living/dead) to provide cell viability as a percentage of total cells. Estimated cell count was determined by the formula:

$$\frac{Viable\ cells}{mL} = \frac{\#\ viable\ cells}{\#\ grids\ counted} * dilution\ factor * 10^4$$

MTT Assay

In addition to Trypan Blue exclusion, experiments involving the quantification of cell viability were conducted by MTT assay. MTT assays measure the reduction of 3-(4,5-Dimethylthiazol-2-yl)-2,5-diphenyltetrazolium bromide in viable cells by action of mitochondrial reductase to a purple formazan crystal. MTT assays (MarkerGene Technologies, Inc., M1475) were carried out in 96-well plates, with each experimental condition repeated 6-fold. Wells around the perimeter of the 96-well plate were not used due to increased risk of evaporation and greater variability experienced in those wells [56]. Once cells were prepared according to the particular experiment, treatments were removed and the cells were washed in 1% PBS. Next, 30μL MTT (2mg/mL) and 170μL HEPES buffer (10mM, pH 7.4) was added to each well and the cells were incubated for 3

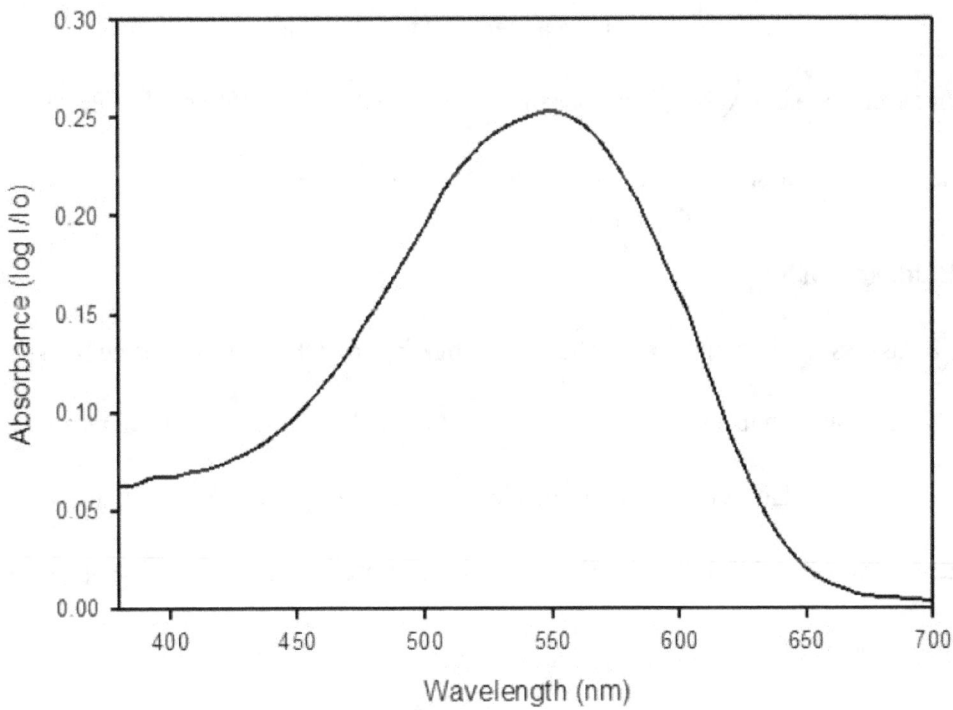

Figure 7. Absorbance spectrum of formazan in dimethyl sulfoxide

25

hours at 37°C and 5% CO_2. Following incubation and visual confirmation of the formation of purple formazan crystals in mock treated wells, the MTT/HEPES solution was carefully aspirated and the crystals were solubilized with 100μL dimethyl sulfoxide. After 15 minutes, the absorbance of each well was read at 570nm (Figure 7) with a background of 620nm in a spectrophotometer with 3 reads per well following 30 seconds of slow orbital rotation and 10 seconds of settling time. Quantitative results are averages of four measurements under the same conditions.

Biocompatibility of AgNPs in Vero cells

The biocompatibility of silver nanoparticles versus silver ions were determined through MTT assay. Vero cells were seeded at $2x10^4$ cells/well in a 96-well plate in DMEM-10 and incubated at 37°C and 5% CO_2. The cells were allowed to stabilize for 24 hours under these conditions prior to treatment. After 24 hours, the cells were exposed to AgNP or silver nitrate ($AgNO_3$) in concentrations of 100μg/mL, 50μg/mL, and 10μg/mL, for 24 hours. MTT assay was performed as described above.

Virus Binding Study

To assess the influence of AgNP in the binding of DENV to target cells, a cold-binding study was conducted. The first steps in the viral life cycle are binding to a target cells and entry into that cell by virus-dependent mechanisms. DENV is able to undergo cell-binding events at 4°C but entry (by clatherin-mediated endocytosis) is not permitted at this low temperature.

Vero cells were seeded at 3×10^4 cells/well in a 12-well μ-slide (Ibidi$^{(R)}$) for 24 hours. Experimental treatments (AgNP-DENV, DENV, and AgNP) were prepared at room temperature for one hour. The AgNP-treated DENV treatment was co-incubated for one hour at room temperature to permit binding of AgNP to DENV. Volumes of AgNP and DENV used in the co-incubation were calculated to provide the desired AgNP concentration and DENV multiplicity of infection (MOI). The required virus inoculum was calculated using the formula:

$$\frac{(cells\ per\ well)(MOI)}{(virus\ titer, pfu)} * 1000 \mu L = (innoculum)\mu L$$

Cells and treatments were cooled to 4°C for 15 minutes. The treatments were incubated with cells for one hour at 4°C. Slides were gently rocked every 15 minutes during treatment. Following cold incubation, cells were gently washed three times with PBS (4°C) to remove unbound DENV and/or AgNP. Control cells were also washed in the same manner. Treatments and washes were removed by pouring onto an absorbent towel.[1] Cells were fixed with chilled 4% paraformaldehyde to prevent the internalization of DENV and AgNP. Indirect fluorescence (without Triton-X permeabilization) was performed to visualize the effects of AgNP on DENV binding to target cells.

Cells were washed three times with PBS. Primary antibody was diluted 1:300 per manufacturer specifications and incubated with cells for one hour at 37°C or overnight at 4°C. The primary antibody used was the Anti-Dengue Virus Serotype 2 Antibody, clone 3H5-1 of mouse origin (MAB8702 Chemicon, Hampshire, United Kingdom). As an

---

[1] Vacuum aspiration repeatedly removed cells in early trials

27

isotype control, normal mouse IgG (NI03, Calbiochem®) was added in place of the 3H5 in one well.

Following incubation, the primary antibody was removed and cells were washed three times with chilled PBS. Secondary antibody was diluted and added to cells for one hour at 37ºC or overnight at 4ºC. The secondary antibody was rabbit anti-mouse IgG-FITC. The secondary antibody was removed and cells washed three times with chilled PBS. Cells were counter-stained with Texas Red®-X Phalloidin for 10 minutes to visualize the polymerized F-actin cytoskeleton of the cells. Cells were washed three times with chilled PBS and a cover slip was mounted using Vectashield® H-1500 which contains DAPI (4',6-diamidino-2-phenylindole, blue) for nuclear visualization.

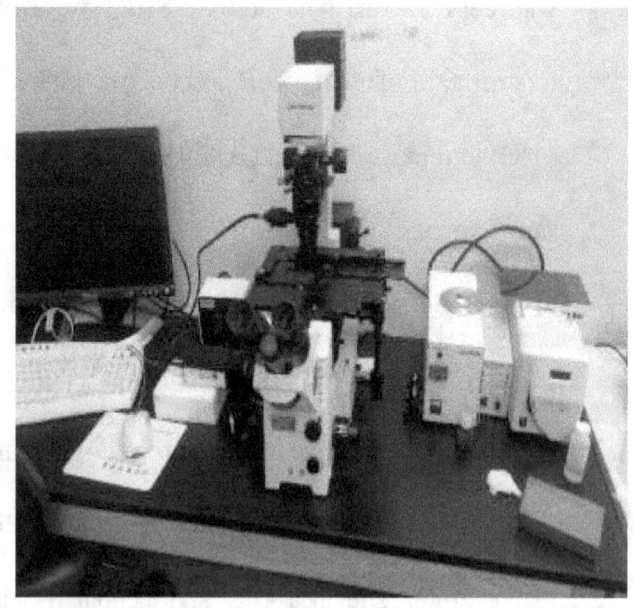

Visualization was performed on an Olympus inverted fluorescence microscope with a CytoViva® Dual Mode Fluorescence system (Figure 8), which provided enhanced visualization of the AgNP. Exposure time required for image capture varied for each fluorescent stain. The optimal values found for these assays were TRITC (tetramethylrhodamine, red) 500ms and FITC (Fluorescein isothiocyanate, green) 1900ms. Optical and software settings were identical when capturing images and not enhanced to artificially increase or decrease fluorescence.

Figure 8. CytoViva Dual Mode Fluorescence System, AI 711th HPW.

Blocking Non-Specific Binding During Immunofluorescence

During indirect immunofluorescence procedures, the decision was made to exclude the common blocking step. Traditionally, cells are incubated with bovine serum albumin (BSA) and serum matching the host of the secondary antibody to block the non-specific binding of antibodies to cell Fc receptors. According to research by Igor Buchwalow, et al, there were no significant differences between various samples that received or did not receive blocking treatment [23]. Buchwalow demonstrated that the standard fixation step removes the ability of endogenous Fc receptors to bind the Fc portion of antibodies. This result was confirmed during early fluorescence trials where blocked and non-blocked samples were compared under the same experimental conditions. In the absence of blocking, background staining was never observed. This decision saved time and lab resources and add further credibility to the suggestion that protein blocking steps, although commonplace in laboratories, are unnecessary.

Image Processing and Analysis

For purposes of this research and the virus binding study, the green (FITC) fluorescent intensity represents the level of DENV attachment to the surface of Vero cells. Image processing methods were used to isolate the fluorescent region of interest (ROI) and remove the background and artifacts. Image analysis methods were used to quantify the differences between ROI. The relative difference in fluorescence intensity between images provided quantifiable differences between the level of DENV binding to cells. Immunofluorescent images were processed and analyzed in ImageJ (National Institutes of Health, http://imagej.nih.gov/ij/). Detailed screenshots of the image processing and analysis steps are contained in Appendix B. Image processing and analysis was conducted using procedures established for the quantification of fluorescence which are accepted within the microscopy community.

The aim of the image processing steps is to isolate the fluorescence that best represents the presence of DENV bound to cell surface receptors. Processing is based on the concept of lookup tables (LUT). Within ImageJ, a color image is converted to an 8-bit image. A single color (green) 8-bit LUT represents 256 possible shades (bins) of green. A LUT value of zero represent black and 255 represents pure green. The fluorescent ROI falls between bins 0-255 but would be impossible to identify with the naked eye. The image processing and analysis steps are described below and summarized in Figure 9:

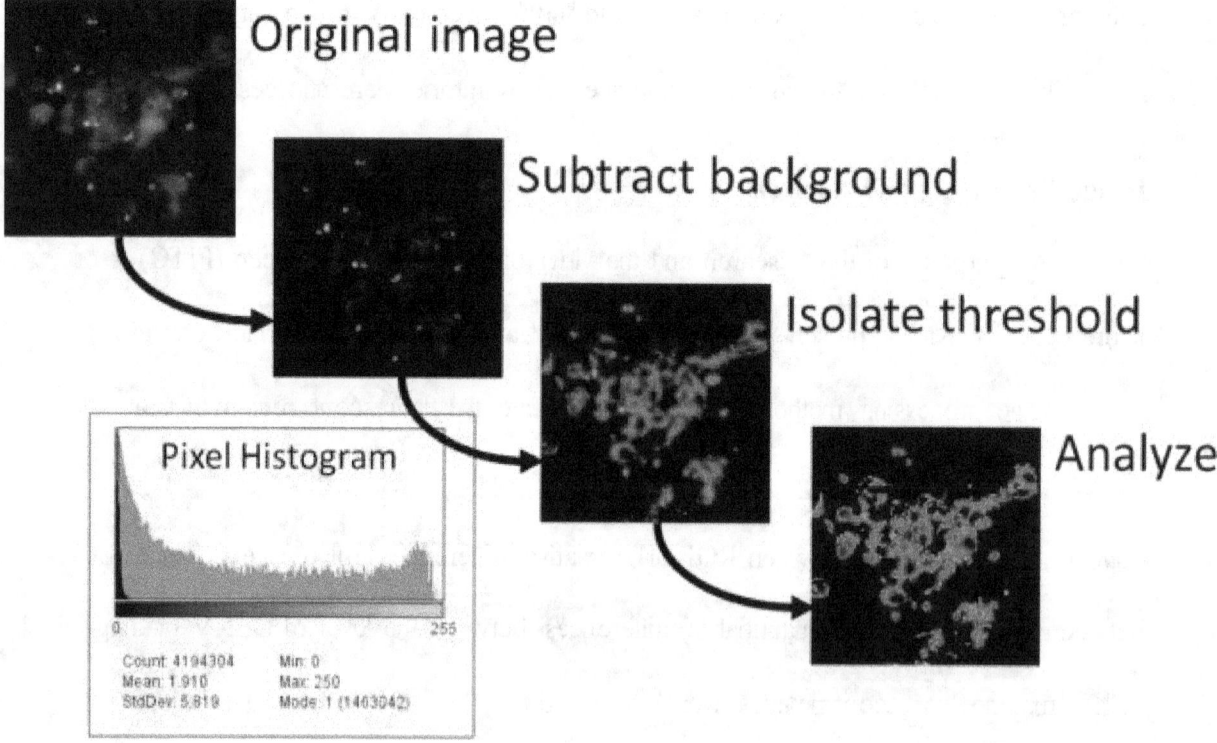

Figure 9. Image processing and analysis overview

30

1.   Convert single-color image to 8-bit. While other image depths are available (i.e. 24-bit, with range 0-4095), the additional resolution is not required for this analysis.

2.   Subtract background. Background subtraction is extremely important when quantifying image intensities. This operation removes constant pixel information from a continuous background (Figure 10). This does not remove the presence of fluorescent artifacts (Figure 11). Artifacts represent areas with high intensity that were not caused by the binding of fluorescently-tagged secondary antibodies to DENV (actually to the primary antibodies bound to DENV E-protein). If artifacts are included in the analysis, they would skew the results and represent greater levels of bound DENV than there truly are.

3.   Identify exclusion regions. Before measuring the fluorescence intensity of an image, the pixel values (bins 0-255) of the exclusion regions must be identified. The two

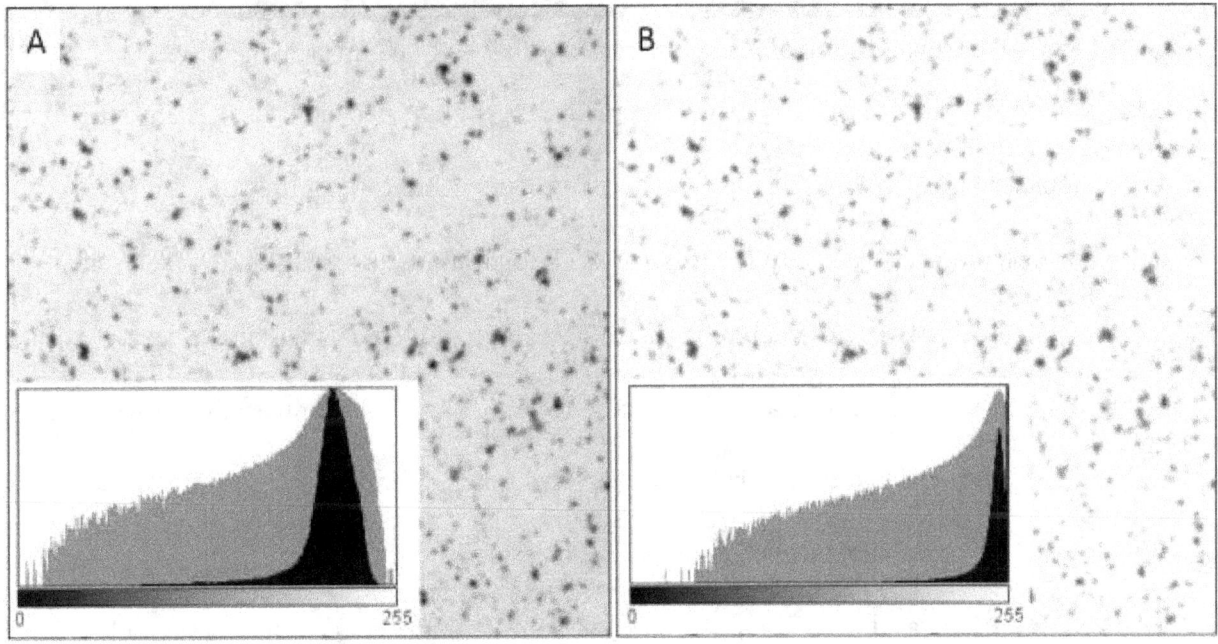

Figure 10. Sample background subtraction in ImageJ. A) Original greyscale image and histogram, B) Image with background subtracted and associated changes to the histogram.

31

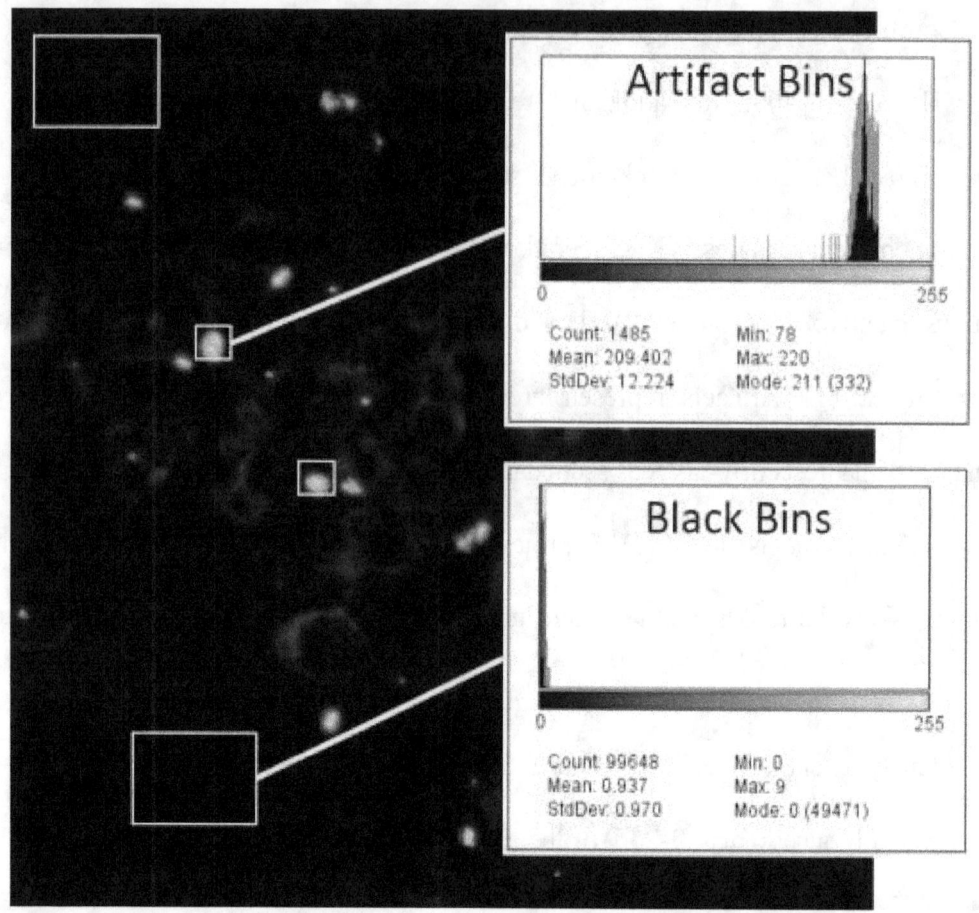

Figure 11. Identification of exclusion regions for black and artifact intensity.

exclusion regions are the black background and the bight, saturated artifacts. The pixel

values representative of these regions are identified through the histograms of selection

areas that only include the area types to exclude. Image histograms graphically represent

the number of occurrences of each pixel value, with each pixel providing one count.

Analyzing the pixel values of black areas far from an ROI will provide the pixel values

representing black background. Analyzing the pixel values of highly saturated artifacts

will provide the pixel values representing false fluorescence intensity that needs to be

excluded from final analysis (Figure 11). Repeated measurements identified that pixel values from 0-8 represent black and values from 198-255 are present only in the artifacts. In each image, the final range of pixel values representing the ROI were bins 9-197.

4.   Isolate the threshold (ROI) using the limits of black maximum and artifact minimum. Within the ImageJ Threshold feature, the pixel values are set to the 9-197 range mentioned above. Thresholding the image to this range creates a binary image where excluded pixels are given a value of 0 and included pixels are given a value of 255. At this point, the image is composed of area that will or will not be included in analysis. This technique does not differentiate between strong fluorescence and weak fluorescence directly, but is used to determine the visible surface area that contains fluorescent values (from original image) determined to be valid intensities. The qualifying area represents the ROI. The thresholding function creates closed objects within which is a portion of the total ROI. Image analysis techniques are next used to measure the total area contained within these ROI "islands" and other properties related to size and distribution.

5.   Analyze images. The target metrics are total ROI area (sq. pixels) and cell count. The Measure Particles function within ImageJ calculates the area of individual ROI islands and provides an image total. Knowing the total area in the image that contained qualifying pixel intensity is required, but does not present the whole story. If the pixel intensity is held constant, an image with more cells should have greater area of ROI. Normalizing an image's ROI area with cell count provides a more accurate estimate of DENV binding per cell. The Cell Counter tool was utilized to count the number of cells in each image. If the normalized region of interest (nROI) is reduced from one image to

the next, it is reasonable to conclude that only the different experimental conditions contributed to the reduction.

RESULTS

Cytotoxicity of DENV Infection of Vero Cells

The effect of DENV infection of Vero cells was analyzed to confirm the infectivity of DENV virus stock and serve as a baseline for virus inhibition studies. Following DENV infection (MOI 0.1), Vero cell viability decreased rapidly from 36-72 hours compared to non-infected cells (Figure 12). By 120hpi, the viability of infected and noninfected cells was comparatively low. Based on visual comparison, the infected cells experienced cytopathic effects and had lifted from the growth surface in patches. The noninfected cells had overgrown and become weakly adherent to the growth surface

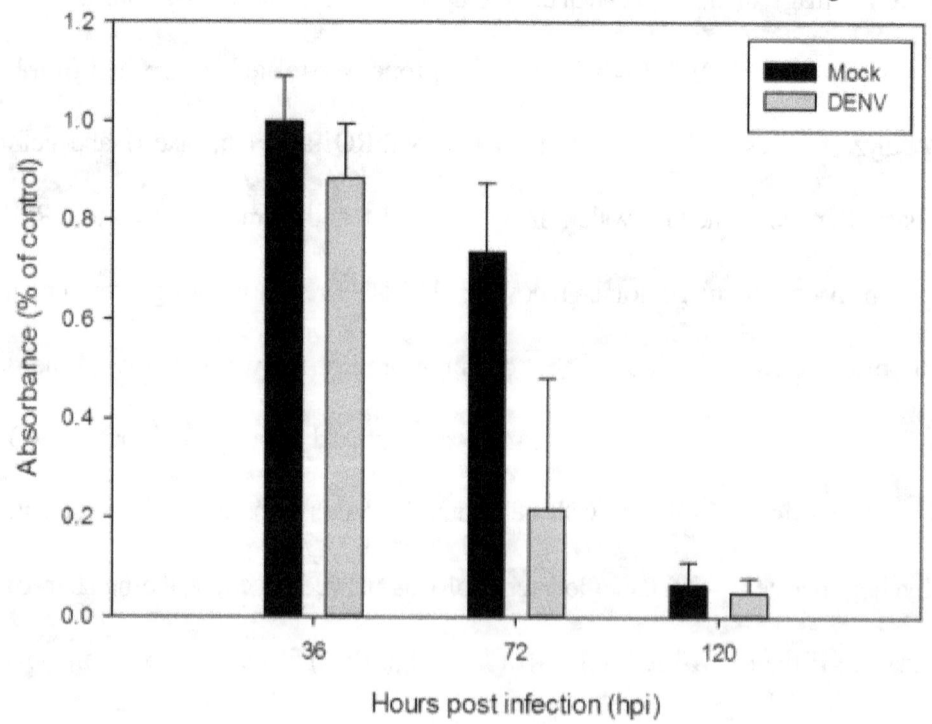

Figure 12. Viability of DENV infected Vero cells.

and were removed from the wells by the gentle force of media aspiration. While the cell viability at 120hpi is similar, it was due to opposing conditions; the Vero cells began to overgrow and die while the DENV infected cells died from infection and lifted from the petri dishes in clusters.

This decline in cell viability was expected, as Vero cells do not have innate defenses against infection. Since Vero cells are highly permissible of DENV infection, they are commonly used to propagate DENV stock during research.

Biocompatibility of AgNPs in Vero cells

Cell viability measured by MTT assay demonstrated that increasing the concentration of AgNP from 10-100μg/mL decreases cell viability relative to mock

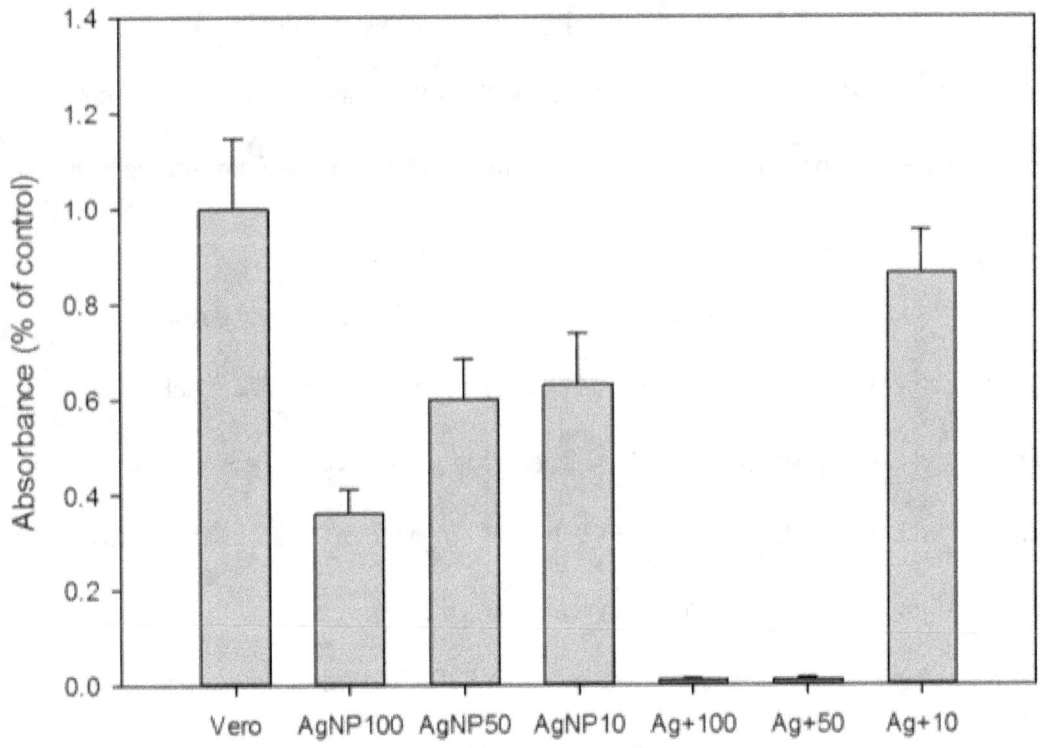

Figure 13. Cytotoxicity of silver nanoparticles (AgNP) versus silver ions (Ag+) at in concentrations of 100μg/mL, 50μg/mL, and 10μg/mL.

treated cells. Positive controls (silver ions, Ag^+) in the same concentrations yielded much greater cytotoxicity than AgNP, with the exception of Ag^+ (10μg/mL), which had higher viability than AgNP. The results suggest that AgNP stock colloid does not have a high concentration of silver ions and that AgNP concentrations should be selected to be as low as possible to minimize cytotoxic effects while providing antiviral or cytoprotective effect from viral infection.

AgNP Inhibition of DENV Binding

Vero cells were incubated with treatments (AgNP-DENV, DENV only, AgNP only) in 4°C to permit binding but inhibit internalization of AgNP and DENV. Based on immunofluorescence analysis, DENV (MOI 40) pretreated with AgNP (25μg/mL), resulted in far fewer bound virion compared to DENV infection without AgNP treatment (positive control) and negative controls (data not shown). Untreated DENV presents greater green fluorescence than after AgNP treatment (Figure 14). Fluorescence images were captured at identical optical and processing software settings.

The reduction in FITC intensity was evaluated in ImageJ as previously described. DENV pretreatment with AgNP (10 and 25μg/mL) reduced fluorescence below the levels of the mock treated and isotype controls (Figure 15). Compared to DENV-only, pretreatment with 10μg/mL reduced DENV binding by a factor of 23.2. Pretreatment with 25μg/mL reduced DENV binding by a factor of 12.2.

Interestingly, the higher concentration of AgNP (25μg/mL) resulted in approximately twice the fluorescence intensity of the lower concentration (10μg/mL). One possible reason this occurred is that higher AgNP concentrations contributed to

36

increased agglomeration. This could reduce the effective number of AgNP available to bind with DENV particles and therefore lead to reduced DENV binding inhibition. Regardless, of the cause of this effect, both AgNP treatments led to fluorescence intensities that were not significantly different than the mock treated control ($P<0.05$).

Comparison of the normalized ROI (nROI) histograms revealed statistically significant differences ($P<0.05$, ANOVA) in the fluorescence intensity of treated cells and controls, and between the AgNP-treated DENV and DENV-only treatments.

While cold incubation does not reflect in vivo conditions during infection, this condition is effective when attempting to isolate the step at which AgNP may inhibit the DENV life cycle. These results are similar to research showing AgNP inhibition of various viruses at the binding and entry phase of viral replication. However, this is the first time a Group IV virus (ss(-)RNA) has been inhibited by AgNP.

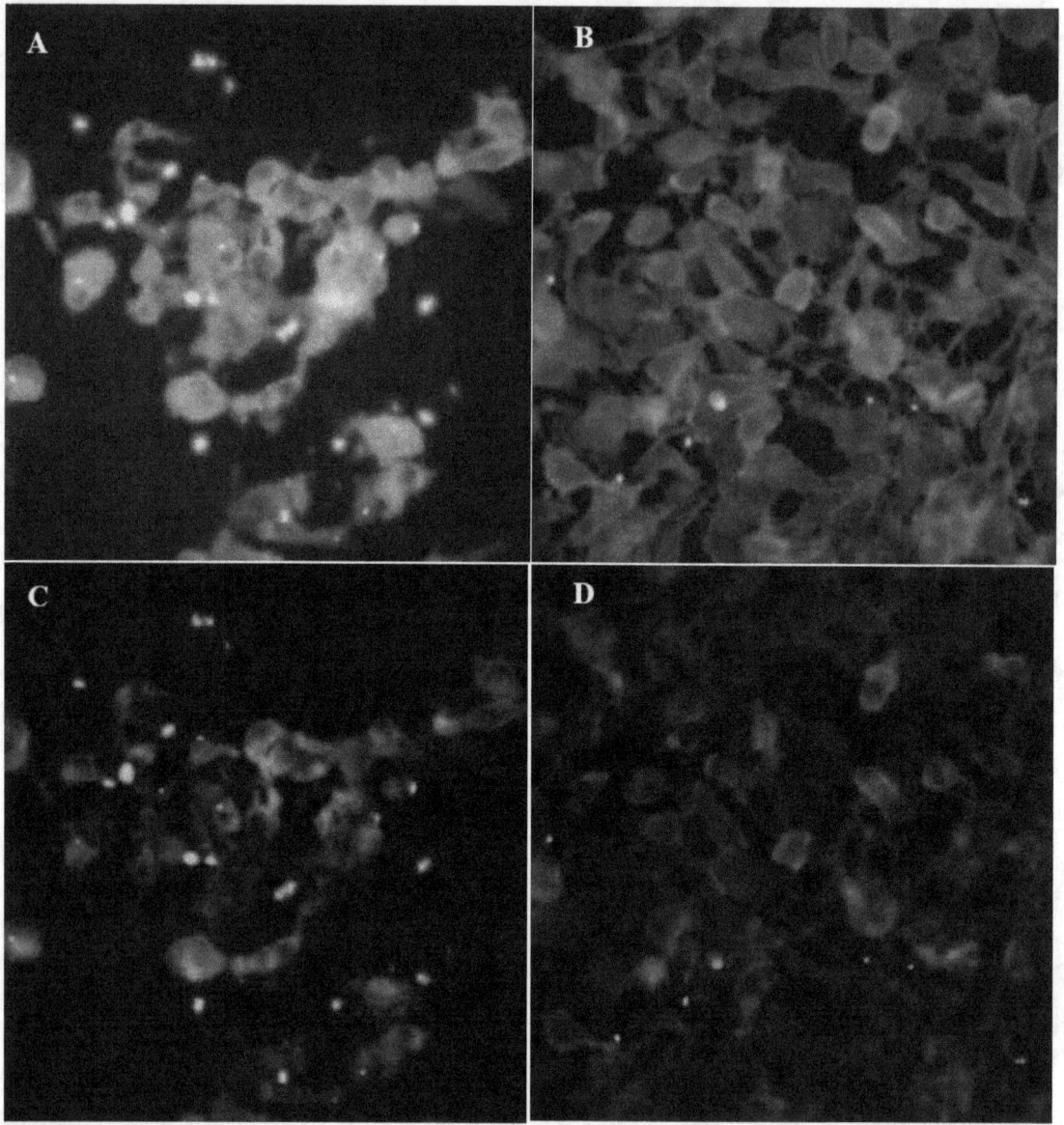

Figure 14. AgNP treatment blocks binding of DENV to Vero cells. (A) DENV binding to Vero cells without AgNP treatment, (B) DENV binding inhibited by pre-treatment with AgNP (25μg/mL). Green fluorescence (FITC, DENV E protein) and red fluorescence (TRITC, f-actin). Image brightness and contrast enhanced 40% for better viewing in print (A & B). (C & D) Non-enhanced composites.

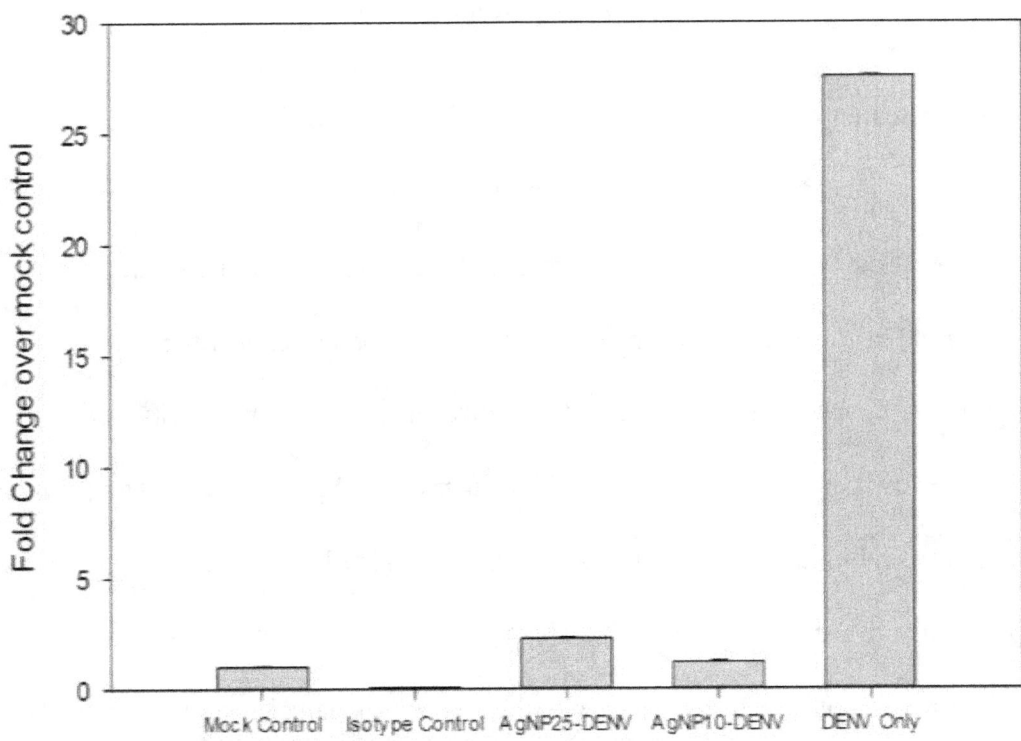

Figure 15. Fluorescence intensity per cell. The isotype control and both AgNP concentrations did not produce fluorescence intensity significantly different from control (P<0.05). DENV-only fluorescence was statistically significant compared to control and both AgNP concentrations (P>0.05).

Statistical Analysis

SigmaPlot 12.0 software (Systat & Mystat Products, Chicago, IL) was used to create graphs and perform statistical analysis. Experimental conditions were compared to mock-treated controls as percent of control. Fluorescent images were also compared to the isotype control to remove the influence of background staining. ImageJ was used to process images as described above.

Histograms representing fluorescence intensities within the ROI were compared using the Mann-Whitney rank sum test. As expected, each histogram failed the normality test (Shapiro-Wilk), therefore, the Mann-Whitney rank sum test provided greater descriptive efficiency than the paired t test.

39

CONCLUSION

This research examined the ability of 8nm silver nanoparticles to inhibit the binding event of dengue virus to Vero cells in vitro. During the course of this research, silver nanoparticles were synthesized, purified, and characterized. Dengue virus type 2 was propagated in Vero cells, quantified and verified for virulence, and purified of bacterial/fungal contaminants. The biocompatibility of AgNP and Vero cells were measured and compared to silver nitrate. The influences of AgNP in the binding event of DENV to Vero cells was visualized through indirect immunofluorescence and quantified through histogram analysis.

The null hypothesis of this study was that silver nanoparticles do not inhibit the binding step of the dengue virus serotype 2 (DENV2) replication cycle in Vero 76 cells, inferred through similar fluorescence intensity visualization. Results indicate that AgNP-pretreated DENV produced a statistically significant reduction in fluorescence intensity compared to DENV infection without AgNP pretreatment ($P<0.05$). Therefore, the null hypothesis is rejected.

This research presents, for the first time that DENV binding to Vero cells is inhibited by 8nm AgNP (citrate stabilized). Fluorescence intensity was 96% (10 μg/mL AgNP) and 92% (25μg/mL AgNP) in AgNP-treated DENV compared to untreated DENV-only infection of Vero cells. A limitation of this study is that the mechanism of binding inhibition is unknown. Existing knowledge on AgNP interaction with viral envelopes suggests that AgNP bind to DENV disulfide regions and possibly others. This could inhibit binding by preventing receptor-epitope covalent interactions. However, it is

40

possible that unbound AgNP in the AgNP-DENV colloid coat the cells and prevent DENV binding in a cytoprotective manner, rather than an antiviral agent.

This serves as a stepping off point for further research into the interaction of AgNP and DENV. Continued research could include:

- Development of a technique to filter unbound AgNP from the AgNP-DENV colloid to prevent unbound AgNP from binding to cells

- Examining the mechanism of binding inhibition by confirming AgNP-DENV binding through TEM/SEM

- Measure cell viability throughout the course of DENV infection versus AgNP-DENV, measured by MTT assay

- Uses of AgNP to disrupt the disease cycle in Aedes mosquitoes

- Progeny virus production following AgNP-treated DENV infection of Vero cells or macrophages, measured by using supernatants from infected cultures to infect second set of cell cultures, quantified by either flow cytometry or MTT assay

- Changes in DENV protein production, measured through Western blot after DENV infection

- Impact of AgNP during DENV infection of macrophages (target cells)

- Quantification of DENV infection after AgNP treatment, measured by flow cytometry

REFERENCES

[1]   A. P. Goncalvez, R. E. Engle, M. St Claire, R. H. Purcell, and C.-J. Lai, "Monoclonal antibody-mediated enhancement of dengue virus infection in vitro and in vivo and strategies for prevention.," *Proc. Natl. Acad. Sci. U. S. A.*, vol. 104, no. 22, pp. 9422–7, May 2007.

[2]   WHO, "Dengue and severe dengue," 2014. [Online]. Available: http://www.who.int/mediacentre/factsheets/fs117/en/.

[3]   CDC, "Dengue Epidemiology," 2014. [Online]. Available: http://www.cdc.gov/dengue/epidemiology/index.html. [Accessed: 09-Jan-2015].

[4]   D. J. Gubler, "Epidemic dengue/dengue hemorrhagic fever as a public health, social and economic problem in the 21st century.," *Trends Microbiol.*, vol. 10, no. 2, pp. 100–3, Mar. 2002.

[5]   E. a Henchal and J. R. Putnak, "The dengue viruses.," *Clin. Microbiol. Rev.*, vol. 3, no. 4, pp. 376–96, Oct. 1990.

[6]   World Health Organization, "Dengue: guidelines for diagnosis, treatment, prevention, and control," *Spec. Program. Res. Train. Trop. Dis.*, pp. x, 147, 2009.

[7]   R. V Gibbons, M. Streitz, T. Babina, and J. R. Fried, "Dengue and US military operations from the Spanish-American War through today.," *Emerg. Infect. Dis.*, vol. 18, no. 4, pp. 623–30, Apr. 2012.

[8]   M. M. Wade, A. E. Chambers, J. M. Insalaco, and A. W. Zulich, "Survival of viral biowarfare agents in disinfected waters.," *Int. J. Microbiol.*, vol. 2010, p. 412694, Jan. 2010.

[9]   J. Hombach, M. Jane Cardosa, A. Sabcharoen, D. W. Vaughn, and A. D. T. Barrett, "Scientific consultation on immunological correlates of protection induced by dengue vaccines. Report from a meeting held at the World Health Organization 17-18 November 2005," in *Vaccine*, 2007, vol. 25, pp. 4130–4139.

[10]   B. L. Innis, K. H. Eckels, E. Kraiselburd, D. R. Dubois, G. F. Meadors, D. J. Gubler, D. S. Burke, and W. H. Bancroft, "Virulence of a live dengue virus vaccine candidate: a possible new marker of dengue virus attenuation.," *J. Infect. Dis.*, vol. 158, pp. 876–880, 1988.

[11]   T. L. Yap, T. Xu, Y.-L. Chen, H. Malet, M.-P. Egloff, B. Canard, S. G. Vasudevan, and J. Lescar, "Crystal structure of the dengue virus RNA-dependent

RNA polymerase catalytic domain at 1.85-angstrom resolution.," *J. Virol.*, vol. 81, no. 9, pp. 4753–65, May 2007.

[12] Z. Yin, Y. Chen, W. Schul, Q. Wang, F. Gu, J. Duraiswamy, W. Liu, B. Liu, J. Y. H. Lim, C. Young, M. Qing, C. Chin, A. Yip, G. Wang, W. Ling, H. Pen, K. Lin, B. Zhang, G. Zou, K. A. Bernard, C. Garrett, K. Beltz, M. Dong, M. Weaver, H. He, A. Pichota, V. Dartois, T. H. Keller, and P. Shi, "An adenosine nucleoside inhibitor of dengue virus," 2009.

[13] A. C. Eifler and C. S. Thaxton, "Nanoparticle therapeutics: FDA approval, clinical trials, regulatory pathways, and case study.," *Methods Mol. Biol.*, vol. 726, pp. 325–38, Jan. 2011.

[14] A. M. Schrand, M. F. Rahman, S. M. Hussain, J. J. Schlager, D. a Smith, and A. F. Syed, "Metal-based nanoparticles and their toxicity assessment.," *Wiley Interdiscip. Rev. Nanomed. Nanobiotechnol.*, vol. 2, no. 5, pp. 544–68, 2010.

[15] R. J. Vandebriel, E. C. Tonk, L. J. de la Fonteyne-Blankestijn, E. R. Gremmer, H. W. Verharen, L. T. van der Ven, H. van Loveren, and W. H. de Jong, "Immunotoxicity of silver nanoparticles in an intravenous 28-day repeated-dose toxicity study in rats.," *Part. Fibre Toxicol.*, vol. 11, no. 1, p. 21, Jan. 2014.

[16] J. S. Kim, J. H. Sung, J. H. Ji, K. S. Song, J. H. Lee, C. S. Kang, and I. J. Yu, "In vivo Genotoxicity of Silver Nanoparticles after 90-day Silver Nanoparticle Inhalation Exposure.," *Saf. Health Work*, vol. 2, no. 1, pp. 34–8, Mar. 2011.

[17] J. H. Lee, Y. S. Kim, K. S. Song, H. R. Ryu, J. H. Sung, J. D. Park, H. M. Park, N. W. Song, B. S. Shin, D. Marshak, K. Ahn, J. E. Lee, and I. J. Yu, "Biopersistence of silver nanoparticles in tissues from Sprague-Dawley rats.," *Part. Fibre Toxicol.*, vol. 10, p. 36, Jan. 2013.

[18] I. Papageorgiou, C. Brown, R. Schins, S. Singh, R. Newson, S. Davis, J. Fisher, E. Ingham, and C. P. Case, "The effect of nano- and micron-sized particles of cobalt-chromium alloy on human fibroblasts in vitro.," *Biomaterials*, vol. 28, no. 19, pp. 2946–58, Jul. 2007.

[19] L. Schnirring, "Researchers identify fifth dengue serotype," *CIDRAP News*, 2013. [Online]. Available: http://www.cidrap.umn.edu/news-perspective/2013/10/researchers-identify-fifth-dengue-subtype.

[20] C. Moore, "UTMB Galveston Researchers Discover First New Dengue Fever Serotype In 50 Years," *BioNews Texas*, 2013. [Online]. Available: http://bionews-tx.com/news/2013/10/25/utmb-galveston-researchers-discover-first-new-dengue-fever-serotype-in-50-years/.

[21]   J. M. da Silva Voorham, "A possible fifth dengue virus serotype," *Ned. Tijdschr. Geneeskd.*, vol. 158, p. A7946, Jan. 2014.

[22]   M. G. Guzmán and G. Kourí, "Dengue: an update.," *Lancet. Infect. Dis.*, vol. 2, no. 1, pp. 33–42, Jan. 2002.

[23]   J. Blok, "Genetic Relationships of the Dengue Virus Serotypes," pp. 1323–1325, 1985.

[24]   R. J. Kuhn, W. Zhang, M. G. Rossmann, S. V Pletnev, J. Corver, E. Lenches, C. T. Jones, S. Mukhopadhyay, P. R. Chipman, E. G. Strauss, T. S. Baker, and J. H. Strauss, "Structure of dengue virus: implications for flavivirus organization, maturation, and fusion.," *Cell*, vol. 108, no. 5, pp. 717–25, Mar. 2002.

[25]   Y. Modis, S. Ogata, D. Clements, and S. C. Harrison, "A ligand-binding pocket in the dengue virus envelope glycoprotein.," *Proc. Natl. Acad. Sci. U. S. A.*, vol. 100, no. 12, pp. 6986–91, Jun. 2003.

[26]   F. Medina, J. F. Medina, C. Colón, E. Vergne, G. A. Santiago, and J. L. Muñoz-Jordán, "Dengue virus: isolation, propagation, quantification, and storage.," *Curr. Protoc. Microbiol.*, vol. Chapter 15, no. November, p. Unit 15D.2., Nov. 2012.

[27]   K. I. P. J. Hidari and T. Suzuki, "Dengue virus receptor.," *Trop. Med. Health*, vol. 39, no. 4 Suppl, pp. 37–43, Dec. 2011.

[28]   J. L. Miller, B. J. de Wet, L. Martinez-Pomares, C. M. Radcliffe, R. a Dwek, P. M. Rudd, and S. Gordon, "The mannose receptor mediates dengue virus infection of macrophages," *PLoS Pathog*, vol. 4, no. 2, p. e17, Feb. 2008.

[29]   J. D. J. Marti, R. M. Angel, and S. Marti, "Identification of a Putative Coreceptor on Vero Cells That Participates in Dengue 4 Virus Infection Identification of a Putative Coreceptor on Vero Cells That Participates in Dengue 4 Virus Infection," vol. 75, no. 17, 2001.

[30]   H. M. van der Schaar, M. J. Rust, C. Chen, H. van der Ende-Metselaar, J. Wilschut, X. Zhuang, and J. M. Smit, "Dissecting the cell entry pathway of dengue virus by single-particle tracking in living cells.," *PLoS Pathog.*, vol. 4, no. 12, p. e1000244, Dec. 2008.

[31]   L. Suksanpaisan, T. Susantad, and D. R. Smith, "Characterization of dengue virus entry into HepG2 cells.," *J. Biomed. Sci.*, vol. 16, no. strain 16007, p. 17, Jan. 2009.

[32] M. N. Krishnan, B. Sukumaran, U. Pal, H. Agaisse, J. L. Murray, T. W. Hodge, and E. Fikrig, "Rab 5 is required for the cellular entry of dengue and West Nile viruses.," *J. Virol.*, vol. 81, no. 9, pp. 4881–5, May 2007.

[33] J. C. Trefry, "The development of silver nanoparticles as antiviral agents," Dayton, 2011.

[34] J. V. Rogers, C. V. Parkinson, Y. W. Choi, J. L. Speshock, and S. M. Hussain, "A Preliminary Assessment of Silver Nanoparticle Inhibition of Monkeypox Virus Plaque Formation," *Nanoscale Res. Lett.*, vol. 3, no. 4, pp. 129–133, Apr. 2008.

[35] E. A. Sopova, V. I. Baranov, O. A. Gankovskaia, V. F. Lavrov, and V. V Zverev, "Effects of silver and silicon dioxide nanopowders on the development of herpesvirus infection in vitro," *Gig. Sanit.*, pp. 89–91.

[36] D. Xiang, Q. Chen, L. Pang, and C. Zheng, "Inhibitory effects of silver nanoparticles on H1N1 influenza A virus in vitro.," *J. Virol. Methods*, vol. 178, no. 1–2, pp. 137–42, Dec. 2011.

[37] D. Xiang, Y. Zheng, W. Duan, X. Li, J. Yin, S. Shigdar, M. L. O'Connor, M. Marappan, X. Zhao, Y. Miao, B. Xiang, and C. Zheng, "Inhibition of A/Human/Hubei/3/2005 (H3N2) influenza virus infection by silver nanoparticles in vitro and in vivo," *Int. J. Nanomedicine*, vol. 8, pp. 4103–4114, 2013.

[38] J. L. Speshock, R. C. Murdock, L. K. Braydich-Stolle, A. M. Schrand, and S. M. Hussain, "Interaction of silver nanoparticles with Tacaribe virus.," *J. Nanobiotechnology*, vol. 8, p. 19, Jan. 2010.

[39] L. Sun, A. K. Singh, K. Vig, S. R. Pillai, and S. R. Singh, "Silver nanoparticles inhibit replication of respiratory syncytial virus," *J. Biomed. Nanotechnol.*, vol. 4, no. 2, pp. 149–158, 2008.

[40] H. H. Lara, N. V Ayala-Nuñez, L. Ixtepan-Turrent, and C. Rodriguez-Padilla, "Mode of antiviral action of silver nanoparticles against HIV-1.," *J. Nanobiotechnology*, vol. 8, p. 1, Jan. 2010.

[41] H. H. Lara, L. Ixtepan-Turrent, E. N. Garza Treviño, and D. K. Singh, "Use of silver nanoparticles increased inhibition of cell-associated HIV-1 infection by neutralizing antibodies developed against HIV-1 envelope proteins.," *J. Nanobiotechnology*, vol. 9, no. 1, p. 38, Jan. 2011.

[42] J. L. Elechiguerra, J. L. Burt, J. R. Morones, A. Camacho-Bragado, X. Gao, H. H. Lara, and M. J. Yacaman, "Interaction of silver nanoparticles with HIV-1.," *J. Nanobiotechnology*, vol. 3, p. 6, Jan. 2005.

[43] J. C. Trefry and D. P. Wooley, "Rapid assessment of antiviral activity and cytotoxicity of silver nanoparticles using a novel application of the tetrazolium-based colorimetric assay.," *J. Virol. Methods*, vol. 183, no. 1, pp. 19–24, Jul. 2012.

[44] L. Lu, R. W.-Y. Sun, R. Chen, C.-K. Hui, C.-M. Ho, J. M. Luk, G. K. K. Lau, and C.-M. Che, "Silver nanoparticles inhibit hepatitis B virus replication.," *Antivir. Ther.*, vol. 13, no. 2, pp. 253–62, Jan. 2008.

[45] N. Chen, Y. Zheng, J. Yin, X. Li, and C. Zheng, "Inhibitory effects of silver nanoparticles against adenovirus type 3 in vitro," *J. Virol. Methods*, vol. 193, no. 2, pp. 470–477, 2013.

[46] J. R. Furr, A. D. Russell, T. D. Turner, and A. Andrews, "Antibacterial activity of Actisorb Plus, Actisorb and silver nitrate," *J. Hosp. Infect.*, vol. 27, no. 3, pp. 201–208, Jul. 1994.

[47] J. Y. Kim, C. Lee, M. Cho, and J. Yoon, "Enhanced inactivation of E. coli and MS-2 phage by silver ions combined with UV-A and visible light irradiation," *Water Res.*, vol. 42, pp. 356–362, 2008.

[48] R. M. Richards, "Antimicrobial action of silver nitrate.," *Microbios*, vol. 31, pp. 83–91, 1981.

[49] P. Jena, S. Mohanty, R. Mallick, B. Jacob, and A. Sonawane, "Toxicity and antibacterial assessment of chitosan-coated silver nanoparticles on human pathogens and macrophage cells.," *Int. J. Nanomedicine*, vol. 7, pp. 1805–18, Jan. 2012.

[50] C. Levard, B. C. Reinsch, F. M. Michel, C. Oumahi, G. V. Lowry, and G. E. Brown, "Sulfidation processes of PVP-coated silver nanoparticles in aqueous solution: Impact on dissolution rate," *Environ. Sci. Technol.*, vol. 45, pp. 5260–5266, 2011.

[51] N. C. Ammerman, M. Beier-Sexton, and A. F. Azad, "Growth and Maintenance of Vero Cell Lines," *Curr. Protoc. Microbiol.*, no. 11, pp. 1–10, 2008.

[52] T. Matsumura, V. Stollar, and R. W. Schlesinger, "Studies on the nature of dengue viruses," *Virology*, vol. 46, no. 2, pp. 344–355, Nov. 1971.

[53] a T. Nahapetian, J. N. Thomas, and W. G. Thilly, "Optimization of environment for high density Vero cell culture: effect of dissolved oxygen and nutrient supply on cell growth and changes in metabolites.," *J. Cell Sci.*, vol. 81, pp. 65–103, Mar. 1986.

[54]   ATCC, "RAW 264.7 (ATCC ® TIB-71 ^TM) Product Sheet." American Type Culture Collection, 2013.

[55]   C.-C. Liu, S.-C. Lee, M. Butler, and S.-C. Wu, "High genetic stability of dengue virus propagated in MRC-5 cells as compared to the virus propagated in vero cells.," *PLoS One*, vol. 3, no. 3, p. e1810, Jan. 2008.

[56]   M. I. Patel, R. Tuckerman, and Q. Dong, "A Pitfall of the 3-(4,5-dimethylthiazol-2-yl)-5(3-carboxymethonyphenol)-2-(4-sulfophenyl)-2H-tetrazolium (MTS) assay due to evaporation in wells on the edge of a 96 well plate.," *Biotechnol. Lett.*, vol. 27, no. 11, pp. 805–8, Jun. 2005.